A PERSONAL
MEDICAL
HISTORY

PAMELA TAYLOR

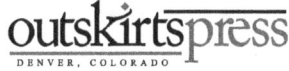

outskirtspress

DENVER, COLORADO

THE PERSONAL MEDICAL HISTORY

OF:

_____

This book is dedicated to my parents,
Vincent and Carrie.

This comprehensive medical log began as sections in a spiral notebook, used by my siblings and me to keep track of the daily vital signs, medication changes, doctor and hospital visits, etc. for our father and mother. The need to keep track of everything became apparent when we started taking Mom and Dad to their doctors' appointments. Before we began the notebook system, we would attempt to piece together information we each had in our aging minds, since we took turns taking Mom and Dad to their appointments.

- When did Dad have those heart stents put in?
- Do you remember why Dad had to go to the emergency room last July and then in November?
- Did anyone bring Dad's Living Will?
- Did Mom receive her flu shot this year?

I hope this log will enable you to monitor and coordinate services for yourself or someone you love. Carry it with you to doctors' appointments, hospital visits, etc. It will also provide useful information to medical emergency personnel at critical times. Your medical history will always be at your fingertips.

TABLE OF CONTENTS

Personal Information

This is the medical history of: _____

Date of Birth: _____

Male: _____   Female: _____

Marital Status: __Single   __Married   __Divorced   __Widowed

Address: _____

_____

_____

Telephone: Home _____

Work _____

Cell _____

Employment Information: _____

_____

_____

_____

MEDICAL DIAGNOSES/ BLOOD TYPE

Medical Diagnoses For: _____

- _____
- _____
- _____
- _____
- _____
- _____
- _____
- _____
- _____
- _____
- _____
- _____

Blood Type: _____

Special Needs: _____

_____

_____

_____

_____

KNOWN ALLERGIES

Known Allergies For: _____

Medication Allergies	Reactions
Other Allergies	

Physicians' Information:

Physician's Name: _____

Specialty Area: _____

Phone Numbers: _____

Address: _____

Physician's Name: _____

Specialty Area: _____

Phone Numbers: _____

Address: _____

Physician's Name: _____

Specialty Area: _____

Phone Numbers: _____

Address: _____

Physician's Name: _____

Specialty Area: _____

Phone Numbers: _____

Address: _____

Physician's Name: _____

Specialty Area: _____

Phone Numbers: _____

Address: _____

Physician's Name: _____

Specialty Area: _____

Phone Numbers: _____

Address: _____

Physicians' Information:

Physician's Name: _____

Specialty Area: _____

Phone Numbers: _____

Address: _____

Physician's Name: _____

Specialty Area: _____

Phone Numbers: _____

Address: _____

Physician's Name: _____

Specialty Area: _____

Phone Numbers: _____

Address: _____

Physician's Name: _____

Specialty Area: _____

Phone Numbers: _____

Address: _____

Physician's Name: _____

Specialty Area: _____

Phone Numbers: _____

Address: _____

Physician's Name: _____

Specialty Area: _____

Phone Numbers: _____

Address: _____

PHYSICIANS' INFORMATION:

Physician's Name: _____

Specialty Area: _____

Phone Numbers: _____

Address: _____

Physician's Name: _____

Specialty Area: _____

Phone Numbers: _____

Address: _____

Physician's Name: _____

Specialty Area: _____

Phone Numbers: _____

Address: _____

Physician's Name: _____

Specialty Area: _____

Phone Numbers: _____

Address: _____

Physician's Name: _____

Specialty Area: _____

Phone Numbers: _____

Address: _____

Physician's Name: _____

Specialty Area: _____

Phone Numbers: _____

Address: _____

EMERGENCY MEDICAL CONTACT INFORMATION

Hospital Preference(s): _____
_____
_____

Ambulance/Transport Services: _____
_____
_____
_____
_____

Pharmacy Preference(s): _____
_____
_____
_____
_____
_____

Other Information: _____
_____
_____
_____
_____
_____
_____
_____
_____
_____
_____

Insurance Information

Insurance Information For: _____

MEDICAL INSURANCE:

Insurance Company	Policy #	Insured's Name	Relationship to Patient

PRESCRIPTION INSURANCE:

Insurance Company	Policy #	Insured's Name	Relationship to Patient

DENTAL INSURANCE:

Insurance Company	Policy #	Insured's Name	Relationship to Patient

INSURANCE INFORMATION

VISION INSURANCE:

Insurance Company	Policy #	Insured's Name	Relationship to Patient

CANCER INSURANCE:

Insurance Company	Policy #	Insured's Name	Relationship to Patient

SHORT-TERM DISABILITY INSURANCE:

Insurance Company	Policy #	Insured's Name	Relationship to Patient

LONG-TERM DISABILITY INSURANCE:

Insurance Company	Policy #	Insured's Name	Relationship to Patient

INSURANCE INFORMATION

LONG-TERM CARE INSURANCE:

Insurance Company	Policy #	Insured's Name	Relationship to Patient

LIFE INSURANCE:

Insurance Company	Policy #	Insured's Name	Relationship to Patient

CAR INSURANCE:

Insurance Company	Policy #	Insured's Name	Relationship to Patient

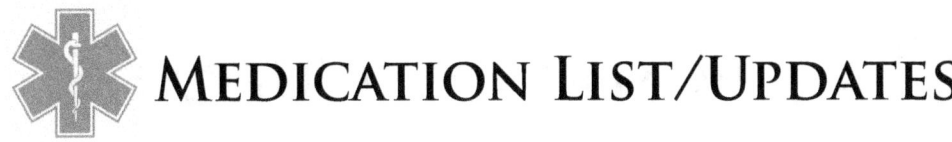

MEDICATION LIST/UPDATES

Medication List For: _____

Date: _____

Name of Medication	Generic Name	Dosage/ Day	Time of Day	Diagnosis/ Reason for Taking	Prescribed By

MEDICATION LIST/UPDATES

Medication List For: _____

Updated On: _____

Name of Medication	Generic Name	Dosage/ Day	Time of Day	Diagnosis/ Reason for Taking	Prescribed By

MEDICATION LIST/UPDATES

Medication List For: _____

Updated On: _____

Name of Medication	Generic Name	Dosage/ Day	Time of Day	Diagnosis/ Reason for Taking	Prescribed By

MEDICATION LIST/UPDATES

Medication List For: _____

Updated On: _____

Name of Medication	Generic Name	Dosage/ Day	Time of Day	Diagnosis/ Reason for Taking	Prescribed By

MEDICATION LIST/UPDATES

Medication List For: _____

Updated On: _____

Name of Medication	Generic Name	Dosage/ Day	Time of Day	Diagnosis/ Reason for Taking	Prescribed By

MEDICATION LIST/UPDATES

Medication List For: _____

Updated On: _____

Name of Medication	Generic Name	Dosage/ Day	Time of Day	Diagnosis/ Reason for Taking	Prescribed By

Medication List/Updates

Medication List For: _____

Updated On: _____

Name of Medication	Generic Name	Dosage/ Day	Time of Day	Diagnosis/ Reason for Taking	Prescribed By

MEDICATION LIST/UPDATES

Medication List For: _____

Updated On: _____

Name of Medication	Generic Name	Dosage/ Day	Time of Day	Diagnosis/ Reason for Taking	Prescribed By

MEDICATION LIST/UPDATES

Medication List For: _____

Updated On: _____

Name of Medication	Generic Name	Dosage/ Day	Time of Day	Diagnosis/ Reason for Taking	Prescribed By

MEDICATION LIST/UPDATES

Medication List For: _____

Updated On: _____

Name of Medication	Generic Name	Dosage/ Day	Time of Day	Diagnosis/ Reason for Taking	Prescribed By

MEDICATION LIST/UPDATES

Medication List For: _____

Updated On: _____

Name of Medication	Generic Name	Dosage/ Day	Time of Day	Diagnosis/ Reason for Taking	Prescribed By

MEDICATION LIST/UPDATES

Medication List For: _____

Updated On: _____

Name of Medication	Generic Name	Dosage/ Day	Time of Day	Diagnosis/ Reason for Taking	Prescribed By

MEDICATION LIST/UPDATES

Medication List For: _____

Updated On: _____

Name of Medication	Generic Name	Dosage/ Day	Time of Day	Diagnosis/ Reason for Taking	Prescribed By

MEDICATION LIST/UPDATES

Medication List For: _____

Updated On: _____

Name of Medication	Generic Name	Dosage/ Day	Time of Day	Diagnosis/ Reason for Taking	Prescribed By

MEDICATION LIST/UPDATES

Medication List For: _____

Updated On: _____

Name of Medication	Generic Name	Dosage/ Day	Time of Day	Diagnosis/ Reason for Taking	Prescribed By

MEDICATION LIST/UPDATES

Medication List For: _____

Updated On: _____

Name of Medication	Generic Name	Dosage/ Day	Time of Day	Diagnosis/ Reason for Taking	Prescribed By

MEDICATION LIST/UPDATES

Medication List For: _____

Updated On: _____

Name of Medication	Generic Name	Dosage/ Day	Time of Day	Diagnosis/ Reason for Taking	Prescribed By

MEDICATION LIST/UPDATES

Medication List For: _____

Updated On: _____

Name of Medication	Generic Name	Dosage/ Day	Time of Day	Diagnosis/ Reason for Taking	Prescribed By

MEDICATION LIST/UPDATES

Medication List For: _____

Updated On: _____

Name of Medication	Generic Name	Dosage/ Day	Time of Day	Diagnosis/ Reason for Taking	Prescribed By

MEDICATION LIST/UPDATES

Medication List For: _____

Updated On: _____

Name of Medication	Generic Name	Dosage/ Day	Time of Day	Diagnosis/ Reason for Taking	Prescribed By

MEDICATION LIST/UPDATES

Medication List For: _____

Updated On: _____

Name of Medication	Generic Name	Dosage/ Day	Time of Day	Diagnosis/ Reason for Taking	Prescribed By

MEDICATION LIST/UPDATES

Medication List For: _____

Updated On: _____

Name of Medication	Generic Name	Dosage/ Day	Time of Day	Diagnosis/ Reason for Taking	Prescribed By

MEDICATION LIST/UPDATES

Medication List For: _____

Updated On: _____

Name of Medication	Generic Name	Dosage/ Day	Time of Day	Diagnosis/ Reason for Taking	Prescribed By

EMERGENCY CONTACT INFORMATION

Name of Contact   Relationship   Phone #s

_____   _____

Home _____

Work _____

Cell _____

Name of Contact   Relationship   Phone #s

_____   _____

Home _____

Work _____

Cell _____

Name of Contact   Relationship   Phone #s

_____   _____

Home _____

Work _____

Cell _____

Name of Contact   Relationship   Phone #s

_____   _____

Home _____

Work _____

Cell _____

Name of Contact   Relationship   Phone #s

_____   _____

Home _____

Work _____

Cell _____

Name of Contact   Relationship   Phone #s

_____   _____

Home _____

Work _____

Cell _____

EMERGENCY CONTACT INFORMATION

Name of Contact   Relationship   Phone #s

_____   _____
Home _____
Work _____
Cell _____

Name of Contact   Relationship   Phone #s

_____   _____
Home _____
Work _____
Cell _____

Name of Contact   Relationship   Phone #s

_____   _____
Home _____
Work _____
Cell _____

Name of Contact   Relationship   Phone #s

_____   _____
Home _____
Work _____
Cell _____

Name of Contact   Relationship   Phone #s

_____   _____
Home _____
Work _____
Cell _____

Name of Contact   Relationship   Phone #s

_____   _____
Home _____
Work _____
Cell _____

EMERGENCY CONTACT INFORMATION

Name of Contact   Relationship   Phone #s

_____   _____   Home _____

Work _____

Cell _____

Name of Contact   Relationship   Phone #s

_____   _____   Home _____

Work _____

Cell _____

Name of Contact   Relationship   Phone #s

_____   _____   Home _____

Work _____

Cell _____

Name of Contact   Relationship   Phone #s

_____   _____   Home _____

Work _____

Cell _____

Name of Contact   Relationship   Phone #s

_____   _____   Home _____

Work _____

Cell _____

Name of Contact   Relationship   Phone #s

_____   _____   Home _____

Work _____

Cell _____

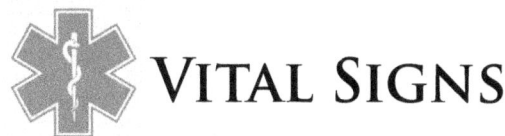

VITAL SIGNS

Vital Signs' Log For: _____

Date / Time	Blood Pressure	Heart Rate	Glucose Reading	Oxygen Level	Temperature

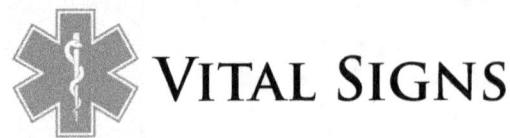

VITAL SIGNS

Vital Signs' Log For: _____

Date / Time	Blood Pressure	Heart Rate	Glucose Reading	Oxygen Level	Temperature

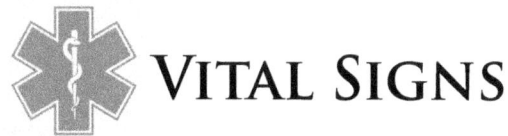

VITAL SIGNS

Vital Signs' Log For: _____

Date / Time	Blood Pressure	Heart Rate	Glucose Reading	Oxygen Level	Temperature

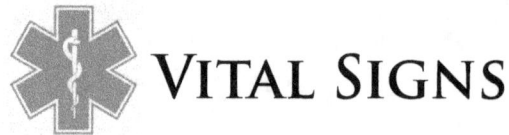

VITAL SIGNS

Vital Signs' Log For: _____

Date / Time	Blood Pressure	Heart Rate	Glucose Reading	Oxygen Level	Temperature

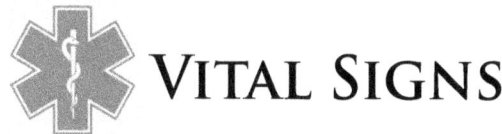

VITAL SIGNS

Vital Signs' Log For: _____

Date / Time	Blood Pressure	Heart Rate	Glucose Reading	Oxygen Level	Temperature

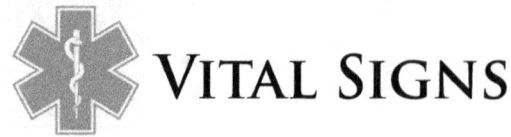

VITAL SIGNS

Vital Signs' Log For: _____

Date / Time	Blood Pressure	Heart Rate	Glucose Reading	Oxygen Level	Temperature

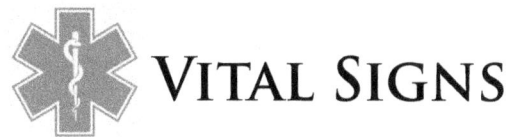

VITAL SIGNS

Vital Signs' Log For: _____

Date / Time	Blood Pressure	Heart Rate	Glucose Reading	Oxygen Level	Temperature

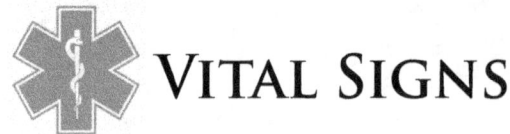

VITAL SIGNS

Vital Signs' Log For: _____

Date / Time	Blood Pressure	Heart Rate	Glucose Reading	Oxygen Level	Temperature

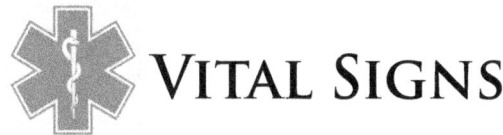

VITAL SIGNS

Vital Signs' Log For: _____

Date / Time	Blood Pressure	Heart Rate	Glucose Reading	Oxygen Level	Temperature

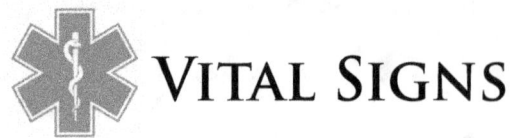

VITAL SIGNS

Vital Signs' Log For: _____

Date / Time	Blood Pressure	Heart Rate	Glucose Reading	Oxygen Level	Temperature

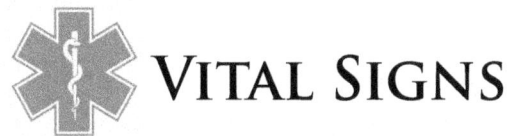

VITAL SIGNS

Vital Signs' Log For: _____

Date / Time	Blood Pressure	Heart Rate	Glucose Reading	Oxygen Level	Temperature

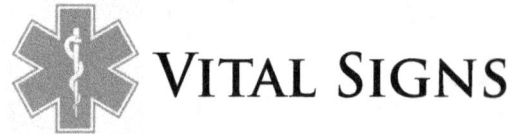

VITAL SIGNS

Vital Signs' Log For: _____

Date / Time	Blood Pressure	Heart Rate	Glucose Reading	Oxygen Level	Temperature

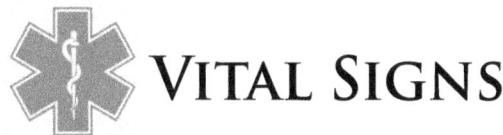

VITAL SIGNS

Vital Signs' Log For: _____

Date / Time	Blood Pressure	Heart Rate	Glucose Reading	Oxygen Level	Temperature

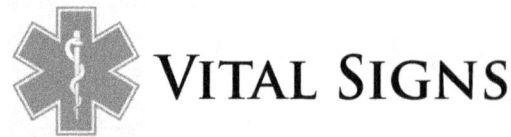

VITAL SIGNS

Vital Signs' Log For: _____

Date / Time	Blood Pressure	Heart Rate	Glucose Reading	Oxygen Level	Temperature

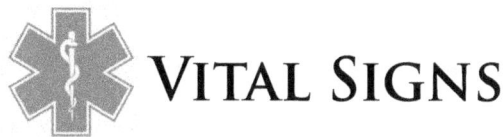
VITAL SIGNS

Vital Signs' Log For: _____

Date / Time	Blood Pressure	Heart Rate	Glucose Reading	Oxygen Level	Temperature

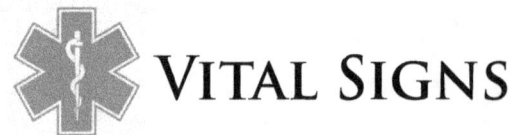

VITAL SIGNS

Vital Signs' Log For: _____

Date / Time	Blood Pressure	Heart Rate	Glucose Reading	Oxygen Level	Temperature

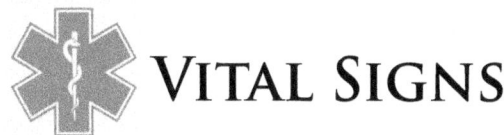

VITAL SIGNS

Vital Signs' Log For: _____

Date / Time	Blood Pressure	Heart Rate	Glucose Reading	Oxygen Level	Temperature

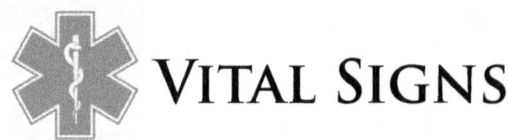

VITAL SIGNS

Vital Signs' Log For: _____

Date / Time	Blood Pressure	Heart Rate	Glucose Reading	Oxygen Level	Temperature

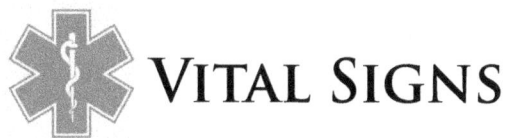

VITAL SIGNS

Vital Signs' Log For: _____

Date / Time	Blood Pressure	Heart Rate	Glucose Reading	Oxygen Level	Temperature

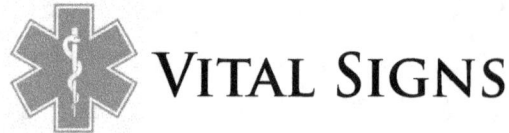

VITAL SIGNS

Vital Signs' Log For: _____

Date / Time	Blood Pressure	Heart Rate	Glucose Reading	Oxygen Level	Temperature

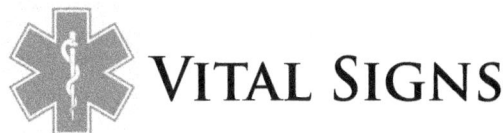

VITAL SIGNS

Vital Signs' Log For: _____

Date / Time	Blood Pressure	Heart Rate	Glucose Reading	Oxygen Level	Temperature

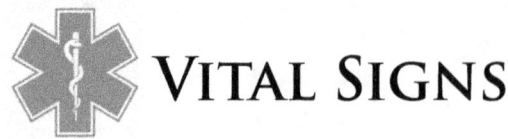

VITAL SIGNS

Vital Signs' Log For: _____

Date / Time	Blood Pressure	Heart Rate	Glucose Reading	Oxygen Level	Temperature

Food/Exercise Log

Date	Exercise	Breakfast	Lunch	Dinner

Food/Exercise Log

Date	Exercise	Breakfast	Lunch	Dinner

FOOD/EXERCISE LOG

Date	Exercise	Breakfast	Lunch	Dinner

Food/Exercise Log

Date	Exercise	Breakfast	Lunch	Dinner

Food/Exercise Log

Date	Exercise	Breakfast	Lunch	Dinner

FOOD/EXERCISE LOG

Date	Exercise	Breakfast	Lunch	Dinner

Food/Exercise Log

Date	Exercise	Breakfast	Lunch	Dinner

FOOD/EXERCISE LOG

Date	Exercise	Breakfast	Lunch	Dinner

Food/Exercise Log

Date	Exercise	Breakfast	Lunch	Dinner

Food/Exercise Log

Date	Exercise	Breakfast	Lunch	Dinner

SHOTS/ VACCINES

Shots' and Vaccines' Record For: _____

Date	Shot/Vaccine Received	Comments

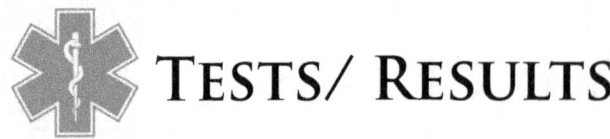

TESTS/ RESULTS

Tests/ Results For: _____

Date	Test(s) Administered	Results

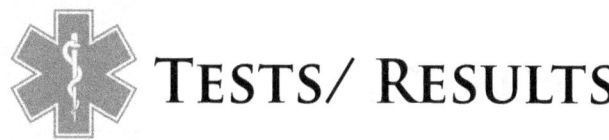

TESTS/ RESULTS

Tests/ Results For: _____

Date	Test(s) Administered	Results

SURGICAL HISTORY

Surgical History For _____

Date	Surgery	Surgeon/ Doctor	Hospital	Comments

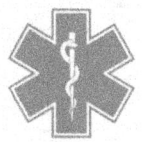

Doctors' Appointments and Notes For:

_____

Date: _____ Appointment with: _____

Reason for visit: _____
_____

Notes: _____
_____
_____
_____
_____
_____
_____
_____

Date: _____ Appointment with: _____

Reason for visit: _____
_____

Notes: _____
_____
_____
_____
_____
_____
_____

Date: _____ Appointment with: _____

Reason for visit: _____

_____

Notes: _____

_____

_____

_____

_____

_____

_____

_____

Date: _____ Appointment with: _____

Reason for visit: _____

_____

Notes: _____

_____

_____

_____

_____

_____

_____

Date: _____ Appointment with: _____

Reason for visit: _____

_____

Notes: _____

_____

_____

_____

_____

_____

_____

_____

Date: _____ Appointment with: _____

Reason for visit: _____

_____

Notes: _____

_____

_____

_____

_____

_____

_____

Date: _____ Appointment with: _____

Reason for visit: _____
_____

Notes: _____
_____
_____
_____
_____
_____
_____
_____
_____

Date: _____ Appointment with: _____

Reason for visit: _____
_____

Notes: _____
_____
_____
_____
_____
_____
_____
_____

Date: _____ Appointment with: _____

Reason for visit: _____

_____

Notes: _____

_____

_____

_____

_____

_____

_____

_____

_____

Date: _____ Appointment with: _____

Reason for visit: _____

_____

Notes: _____

_____

_____

_____

_____

_____

_____

_____

Date: _____ Appointment with: _____

Reason for visit: _____

_____

Notes: _____

_____

_____

_____

_____

_____

_____

_____

Date: _____ Appointment with: _____

Reason for visit: _____

_____

Notes: _____

_____

_____

_____

_____

_____

_____

Date: _____ Appointment with: _____

Reason for visit: _____
_____

Notes: _____
_____
_____
_____
_____
_____
_____
_____
_____

Date: _____ Appointment with: _____

Reason for visit: _____
_____

Notes: _____
_____
_____
_____
_____
_____
_____
_____

Date: _____ Appointment with: _____

Reason for visit: _____

_____

Notes: _____

_____

_____

_____

_____

_____

_____

_____

Date: _____ Appointment with: _____

Reason for visit: _____

_____

Notes: _____

_____

_____

_____

_____

_____

_____

_____

Date: _____ Appointment with: _____

Reason for visit: _____
_____

Notes: _____
_____
_____
_____
_____
_____
_____
_____

Date: _____ Appointment with: _____

Reason for visit: _____
_____

Notes: _____
_____
_____
_____
_____
_____
_____
_____

Date: _____ Appointment with: _____

Reason for visit: _____

_____

Notes: _____

_____

_____

_____

_____

_____

_____

_____

_____

Date: _____ Appointment with: _____

Reason for visit: _____

_____

Notes: _____

_____

_____

_____

_____

_____

_____

_____

Date: _____ Appointment with: _____

Reason for visit: _____
_____

Notes: _____
_____
_____
_____
_____
_____
_____
_____
_____

Date: _____ Appointment with: _____

Reason for visit: _____
_____

Notes: _____
_____
_____
_____
_____
_____
_____
_____

Date: _____ Appointment with: _____

Reason for visit: _____

_____

Notes: _____

_____

_____

_____

_____

_____

_____

_____

_____

Date: _____ Appointment with: _____

Reason for visit: _____

_____

Notes: _____

_____

_____

_____

_____

_____

_____

_____

Date: _____ Appointment with: _____

Reason for visit: _____

_____

Notes: _____

_____

_____

_____

_____

_____

_____

_____

Date: _____ Appointment with: _____

Reason for visit: _____

_____

Notes: _____

_____

_____

_____

_____

_____

_____

_____

Date: _____ Appointment with: _____

Reason for visit: _____

_____

Notes: _____

_____

_____

_____

_____

_____

_____

_____

Date: _____ Appointment with: _____

Reason for visit: _____

_____

Notes: _____

_____

_____

_____

_____

_____

_____

Date: _____ Appointment with: _____

Reason for visit: _____
_____

Notes: _____
_____
_____
_____
_____
_____
_____
_____
_____
_____

Date: _____ Appointment with: _____

Reason for visit: _____
_____

Notes: _____
_____
_____
_____
_____
_____
_____
_____

Date: _____ Appointment with: _____

Reason for visit: _____

_____

Notes: _____

_____

_____

_____

_____

_____

_____

_____

_____

_____

Date: _____ Appointment with: _____

Reason for visit: _____

_____

Notes: _____

_____

_____

_____

_____

_____

_____

_____

Date: _____ Appointment with: _____

Reason for visit: _____
_____

Notes: _____
_____
_____
_____
_____
_____
_____
_____

Date: _____ Appointment with: _____

Reason for visit: _____
_____

Notes: _____
_____
_____
_____
_____
_____
_____
_____

Date: _____ Appointment with: _____

Reason for visit: _____
_____

Notes: _____
_____
_____
_____
_____
_____
_____
_____
_____

Date: _____ Appointment with: _____

Reason for visit: _____
_____

Notes: _____
_____
_____
_____
_____
_____
_____
_____

Date: _____ Appointment with: _____

Reason for visit: _____
_____

Notes: _____
_____
_____
_____
_____
_____
_____
_____
_____

Date: _____ Appointment with: _____

Reason for visit: _____
_____

Notes: _____
_____
_____
_____
_____
_____
_____
_____

Date: _____ Appointment with: _____

Reason for visit: _____

_____

Notes: _____

_____

_____

_____

_____

_____

_____

_____

Date: _____ Appointment with: _____

Reason for visit: _____

_____

Notes: _____

_____

_____

_____

_____

_____

_____

_____

Date: _____ Appointment with: _____

Reason for visit: _____
_____

Notes: _____
_____
_____
_____
_____
_____
_____
_____
_____

Date: _____ Appointment with: _____

Reason for visit: _____
_____

Notes: _____
_____
_____
_____
_____
_____
_____
_____

Date: _____ Appointment with: _____

Reason for visit: _____

_____

Notes: _____

_____

_____

_____

_____

_____

_____

_____

_____

Date: _____ Appointment with: _____

Reason for visit: _____

_____

Notes: _____

_____

_____

_____

_____

_____

_____

_____

Date: _____ Appointment with: _____

Reason for visit: _____

_____

Notes: _____

_____

_____

_____

_____

_____

_____

_____

_____

Date: _____ Appointment with: _____

Reason for visit: _____

_____

Notes: _____

_____

_____

_____

_____

_____

_____

_____

Date: _____ Appointment with: _____

Reason for visit: _____
_____

Notes: _____
_____
_____
_____
_____
_____
_____
_____
_____

Date: _____ Appointment with: _____

Reason for visit: _____
_____

Notes: _____
_____
_____
_____
_____
_____
_____
_____

Date: _____ Appointment with: _____

Reason for visit: _____
_____

Notes: _____
_____
_____
_____
_____
_____
_____
_____
_____

Date: _____ Appointment with: _____

Reason for visit: _____
_____

Notes: _____
_____
_____
_____
_____
_____
_____
_____

Date: _____ Appointment with: _____

Reason for visit: _____

_____

Notes: _____

_____

_____

_____

_____

_____

_____

_____

Date: _____ Appointment with: _____

Reason for visit: _____

_____

Notes: _____

_____

_____

_____

_____

_____

_____

_____

Date: _____ Appointment with: _____

Reason for visit: _____

_____

Notes: _____

_____

_____

_____

_____

_____

_____

_____

_____

Date: _____ Appointment with: _____

Reason for visit: _____

_____

Notes: _____

_____

_____

_____

_____

_____

_____

_____

Date: _____ Appointment with: _____

Reason for visit: _____

_____

Notes: _____

_____

_____

_____

_____

_____

_____

_____

_____

Date: _____ Appointment with: _____

Reason for visit: _____

_____

Notes: _____

_____

_____

_____

_____

_____

_____

_____

Date: _____ Appointment with: _____

Reason for visit: _____

_____

Notes: _____

_____

_____

_____

_____

_____

_____

_____

_____

Date: _____ Appointment with: _____

Reason for visit: _____

_____

Notes: _____

_____

_____

_____

_____

_____

_____

_____

Date: _____ Appointment with: _____

Reason for visit: _____
_____

Notes: _____
_____
_____
_____
_____
_____
_____
_____
_____

Date: _____ Appointment with: _____

Reason for visit: _____
_____

Notes: _____
_____
_____
_____
_____
_____
_____
_____

Date: _____ Appointment with: _____

Reason for visit: _____

_____

Notes: _____

_____

_____

_____

_____

_____

_____

_____

_____

Date: _____ Appointment with: _____

Reason for visit: _____

_____

Notes: _____

_____

_____

_____

_____

_____

_____

_____

Date: _____ Appointment with: _____

Reason for visit: _____

_____

Notes: _____

_____

_____

_____

_____

_____

_____

_____

_____

Date: _____ Appointment with: _____

Reason for visit: _____

_____

Notes: _____

_____

_____

_____

_____

_____

_____

_____

Date: _____ Appointment with: _____

Reason for visit: _____

_____

Notes: _____

_____

_____

_____

_____

_____

_____

_____

_____

Date: _____ Appointment with: _____

Reason for visit: _____

_____

Notes: _____

_____

_____

_____

_____

_____

_____

_____

Date: _____ Appointment with: _____

Reason for visit: _____

_____

Notes: _____

_____

_____

_____

_____

_____

_____

_____

_____

Date: _____ Appointment with: _____

Reason for visit: _____

_____

Notes: _____

_____

_____

_____

_____

_____

_____

_____

Date: _____ Appointment with: _____

Reason for visit: _____

_____

Notes: _____

_____

_____

_____

_____

_____

_____

_____

_____

Date: _____ Appointment with: _____

Reason for visit: _____

_____

Notes: _____

_____

_____

_____

_____

_____

_____

_____

Date: _____ Appointment with: _____

Reason for visit: _____

_____

Notes: _____

_____

_____

_____

_____

_____

_____

_____

_____

Date: _____ Appointment with: _____

Reason for visit: _____

_____

Notes: _____

_____

_____

_____

_____

_____

_____

_____

_____

Date: _____ Appointment with: _____

Reason for visit: _____

_____

Notes: _____

_____

_____

_____

_____

_____

_____

_____

_____

Date: _____ Appointment with: _____

Reason for visit: _____

_____

Notes: _____

_____

_____

_____

_____

_____

_____

_____

Date: _____ Appointment with: _____

Reason for visit: _____

_____

Notes: _____

_____

_____

_____

_____

_____

_____

_____

_____

Date: _____ Appointment with: _____

Reason for visit: _____

_____

Notes: _____

_____

_____

_____

_____

_____

_____

_____

Date: _____ Appointment with: _____

Reason for visit: _____

_____

Notes: _____

_____

_____

_____

_____

_____

_____

_____

_____

Date: _____ Appointment with: _____

Reason for visit: _____

_____

Notes: _____

_____

_____

_____

_____

_____

_____

_____

Date: _____ Appointment with: _____

Reason for visit: _____

_____

Notes: _____

_____

_____

_____

_____

_____

_____

_____

_____

Date: _____ Appointment with: _____

Reason for visit: _____

_____

Notes: _____

_____

_____

_____

_____

_____

_____

_____

Date: _____ Appointment with: _____

Reason for visit: _____

_____

Notes: _____

_____

_____

_____

_____

_____

_____

_____

_____

Date: _____ Appointment with: _____

Reason for visit: _____

_____

Notes: _____

_____

_____

_____

_____

_____

_____

_____

Date: _____ Appointment with: _____

Reason for visit: _____

_____

Notes: _____

_____

_____

_____

_____

_____

_____

_____

Date: _____ Appointment with: _____

Reason for visit: _____

_____

Notes: _____

_____

_____

_____

_____

_____

_____

_____

Date: _____ Appointment with: _____

Reason for visit: _____

_____

Notes: _____

_____

_____

_____

_____

_____

_____

_____

Date: _____ Appointment with: _____

Reason for visit: _____

_____

Notes: _____

_____

_____

_____

_____

_____

_____

Date: _____ Appointment with: _____

Reason for visit: _____

_____

Notes: _____

_____

_____

_____

_____

_____

_____

_____

_____

Date: _____ Appointment with: _____

Reason for visit: _____

_____

Notes: _____

_____

_____

_____

_____

_____

_____

_____

Date: _____ Appointment with: _____

Reason for visit: _____

_____

Notes: _____

_____

_____

_____

_____

_____

_____

_____

Date: _____ Appointment with: _____

Reason for visit: _____

_____

Notes: _____

_____

_____

_____

_____

_____

_____

_____

Date: _____ Appointment with: _____

Reason for visit: _____

_____

Notes: _____

_____

_____

_____

_____

_____

_____

_____

Date: _____ Appointment with: _____

Reason for visit: _____

_____

Notes: _____

_____

_____

_____

_____

_____

_____

_____

Date: _____ Appointment with: _____

Reason for visit: _____

_____

Notes: _____

_____

_____

_____

_____

_____

_____

_____

_____

Date: _____ Appointment with: _____

Reason for visit: _____

_____

Notes: _____

_____

_____

_____

_____

_____

_____

_____

Date: _____ Appointment with: _____

Reason for visit: _____

_____

Notes: _____

_____

_____

_____

_____

_____

_____

_____

_____

Date: _____ Appointment with: _____

Reason for visit: _____

_____

Notes: _____

_____

_____

_____

_____

_____

_____

_____

Date: _____ Appointment with: _____

Reason for visit: _____

_____

Notes: _____

_____

_____

_____

_____

_____

_____

_____

Date: _____ Appointment with: _____

Reason for visit: _____

_____

Notes: _____

_____

_____

_____

_____

_____

_____

Date: _____ Appointment with: _____

Reason for visit: _____

_____

Notes: _____

_____

_____

_____

_____

_____

_____

_____

Date: _____ Appointment with: _____

Reason for visit: _____

_____

Notes: _____

_____

_____

_____

_____

_____

_____

Date: _____ Appointment with: _____

Reason for visit: _____

_____

Notes: _____

_____

_____

_____

_____

_____

_____

_____

_____

Date: _____ Appointment with: _____

Reason for visit: _____

_____

Notes: _____

_____

_____

_____

_____

_____

_____

_____

Date: _____ Appointment with: _____

Reason for visit: _____

_____

Notes: _____

_____

_____

_____

_____

_____

_____

_____

_____

Date: _____ Appointment with: _____

Reason for visit: _____

_____

Notes: _____

_____

_____

_____

_____

_____

_____

_____

Date: _____ Appointment with: _____

Reason for visit: _____
_____

Notes: _____
_____
_____
_____
_____
_____
_____
_____
_____

Date: _____ Appointment with: _____

Reason for visit: _____
_____

Notes: _____
_____
_____
_____
_____
_____
_____
_____

Date: _____ Appointment with: _____

Reason for visit: _____
_____

Notes: _____
_____
_____
_____
_____
_____
_____
_____
_____

Date: _____ Appointment with: _____

Reason for visit: _____
_____

Notes: _____
_____
_____
_____
_____
_____
_____
_____

Date: _____ Appointment with: _____

Reason for visit: _____

_____

Notes: _____

_____

_____

_____

_____

_____

_____

_____

_____

Date: _____ Appointment with: _____

Reason for visit: _____

_____

Notes: _____

_____

_____

_____

_____

_____

_____

_____

Date: _____ Appointment with: _____

Reason for visit: _____

_____

Notes: _____

_____

_____

_____

_____

_____

_____

_____

Date: _____ Appointment with: _____

Reason for visit: _____

_____

Notes: _____

_____

_____

_____

_____

_____

_____

_____

Date: _____ Appointment with: _____

Reason for visit: _____

_____

Notes: _____

_____

_____

_____

_____

_____

_____

_____

Date: _____ Appointment with: _____

Reason for visit: _____

_____

Notes: _____

_____

_____

_____

_____

_____

_____

_____

Date: _____ Appointment with: _____

Reason for visit: _____
_____

Notes: _____
_____
_____
_____
_____
_____
_____
_____
_____

Date: _____ Appointment with: _____

Reason for visit: _____
_____

Notes: _____
_____
_____
_____
_____
_____
_____
_____

Date: _____ Appointment with: _____

Reason for visit: _____
_____

Notes: _____
_____
_____
_____
_____
_____
_____
_____
_____

Date: _____ Appointment with: _____

Reason for visit: _____
_____

Notes: _____
_____
_____
_____
_____
_____
_____
_____

Date: _____ Appointment with: _____

Reason for visit: _____

_____

Notes: _____

_____

_____

_____

_____

_____

_____

_____

_____

Date: _____ Appointment with: _____

Reason for visit: _____

_____

Notes: _____

_____

_____

_____

_____

_____

_____

_____

Date: _____ Appointment with: _____

Reason for visit: _____

_____

Notes: _____

_____

_____

_____

_____

_____

_____

_____

Date: _____ Appointment with: _____

Reason for visit: _____

_____

Notes: _____

_____

_____

_____

_____

_____

_____

_____

Date: _____ Appointment with: _____

Reason for visit: _____

_____

Notes: _____

_____

_____

_____

_____

_____

_____

_____

_____

Date: _____ Appointment with: _____

Reason for visit: _____

_____

Notes: _____

_____

_____

_____

_____

_____

_____

_____

Date: _____ Appointment with: _____

Reason for visit: _____

_____

Notes: _____

_____

_____

_____

_____

_____

_____

_____

_____

Date: _____ Appointment with: _____

Reason for visit: _____

_____

Notes: _____

_____

_____

_____

_____

_____

_____

_____

Date: _____ Appointment with: _____

Reason for visit: _____

_____

Notes: _____

_____

_____

_____

_____

_____

_____

_____

_____

Date: _____ Appointment with: _____

Reason for visit: _____

_____

Notes: _____

_____

_____

_____

_____

_____

_____

_____

Date: _____ Appointment with: _____

Reason for visit: _____

_____

Notes: _____

_____

_____

_____

_____

_____

_____

_____

_____

Date: _____ Appointment with: _____

Reason for visit: _____

_____

Notes: _____

_____

_____

_____

_____

_____

_____

_____

Date: _____ Appointment with: _____

Reason for visit: _____
_____

Notes: _____
_____
_____
_____
_____
_____
_____
_____
_____

Date: _____ Appointment with: _____

Reason for visit: _____
_____

Notes: _____
_____
_____
_____
_____
_____
_____
_____

Date: _____ Appointment with: _____

Reason for visit: _____

_____

Notes: _____

_____

_____

_____

_____

_____

_____

_____

_____

Date: _____ Appointment with: _____

Reason for visit: _____

_____

Notes: _____

_____

_____

_____

_____

_____

_____

_____

Date: _____ Appointment with: _____

Reason for visit: _____

_____

Notes: _____

_____

_____

_____

_____

_____

_____

_____

_____

Date: _____ Appointment with: _____

Reason for visit: _____

_____

Notes: _____

_____

_____

_____

_____

_____

_____

_____

Date: _____ Appointment with: _____

Reason for visit: _____
_____

Notes: _____
_____
_____
_____
_____
_____
_____
_____
_____

Date: _____ Appointment with: _____

Reason for visit: _____
_____

Notes: _____
_____
_____
_____
_____
_____
_____
_____

Date: _____ Appointment with: _____

Reason for visit: _____

_____

Notes: _____

_____

_____

_____

_____

_____

_____

_____

_____

Date: _____ Appointment with: _____

Reason for visit: _____

_____

Notes: _____

_____

_____

_____

_____

_____

_____

_____

Date: _____ Appointment with: _____

Reason for visit: _____

_____

Notes: _____

_____

_____

_____

_____

_____

_____

_____

_____

Date: _____ Appointment with: _____

Reason for visit: _____

_____

Notes: _____

_____

_____

_____

_____

_____

_____

_____

Date: _____ Appointment with: _____

Reason for visit: _____

_____

Notes: _____

_____

_____

_____

_____

_____

_____

_____

_____

Date: _____ Appointment with: _____

Reason for visit: _____

_____

Notes: _____

_____

_____

_____

_____

_____

_____

_____

Date: _____ Appointment with: _____

Reason for visit: _____
_____

Notes: _____
_____
_____
_____
_____
_____
_____
_____
_____

Date: _____ Appointment with: _____

Reason for visit: _____
_____

Notes: _____
_____
_____
_____
_____
_____
_____
_____

Date: _____ Appointment with: _____

Reason for visit: _____

_____

Notes: _____

_____

_____

_____

_____

_____

_____

_____

Date: _____ Appointment with: _____

Reason for visit: _____

_____

Notes: _____

_____

_____

_____

_____

_____

_____

_____

Date: _____ Appointment with: _____

Reason for visit: _____

_____

Notes: _____

_____

_____

_____

_____

_____

_____

_____

_____

Date: _____ Appointment with: _____

Reason for visit: _____

_____

Notes: _____

_____

_____

_____

_____

_____

_____

_____

Date: _____ Appointment with: _____

Reason for visit: _____
_____

Notes: _____
_____
_____
_____
_____
_____
_____
_____
_____

Date: _____ Appointment with: _____

Reason for visit: _____
_____

Notes: _____
_____
_____
_____
_____
_____
_____
_____

Date: _____ Appointment with: _____

Reason for visit: _____

_____

Notes: _____

_____

_____

_____

_____

_____

_____

_____

_____

Date: _____ Appointment with: _____

Reason for visit: _____

_____

Notes: _____

_____

_____

_____

_____

_____

_____

_____

Date: _____ Appointment with: _____

Reason for visit: _____

_____

Notes: _____

_____

_____

_____

_____

_____

_____

_____

_____

Date: _____ Appointment with: _____

Reason for visit: _____

_____

Notes: _____

_____

_____

_____

_____

_____

_____

_____

Date: _____ Appointment with: _____

Reason for visit: _____
_____

Notes: _____
_____
_____
_____
_____
_____
_____
_____
_____

Date: _____ Appointment with: _____

Reason for visit: _____
_____

Notes: _____
_____
_____
_____
_____
_____
_____
_____

Date: _____ Appointment with: _____

Reason for visit: _____

_____

Notes: _____

_____

_____

_____

_____

_____

_____

_____

Date: _____ Appointment with: _____

Reason for visit: _____

_____

Notes: _____

_____

_____

_____

_____

_____

_____

_____

Date: _____ Appointment with: _____

Reason for visit: _____

_____

Notes: _____

_____

_____

_____

_____

_____

_____

_____

Date: _____ Appointment with: _____

Reason for visit: _____

_____

Notes: _____

_____

_____

_____

_____

_____

_____

Date: _____ Appointment with: _____

Reason for visit: _____

_____

Notes: _____

_____

_____

_____

_____

_____

_____

_____

Date: _____ Appointment with: _____

Reason for visit: _____

_____

Notes: _____

_____

_____

_____

_____

_____

_____

_____

Date: _____ Appointment with: _____

Reason for visit: _____

_____

Notes: _____

_____

_____

_____

_____

_____

_____

_____

_____

Date: _____ Appointment with: _____

Reason for visit: _____

_____

Notes: _____

_____

_____

_____

_____

_____

_____

Date: _____ Appointment with: _____

Reason for visit: _____

_____

Notes: _____

_____

_____

_____

_____

_____

_____

_____

_____

Date: _____ Appointment with: _____

Reason for visit: _____

_____

Notes: _____

_____

_____

_____

_____

_____

_____

_____

Date: _____ Appointment with: _____

Reason for visit: _____

_____

Notes: _____

_____

_____

_____

_____

_____

_____

_____

Date: _____ Appointment with: _____

Reason for visit: _____

_____

Notes: _____

_____

_____

_____

_____

_____

_____

Date: _____ Appointment with: _____

Reason for visit: _____
_____

Notes: _____
_____
_____
_____
_____
_____
_____
_____
_____

Date: _____ Appointment with: _____

Reason for visit: _____
_____

Notes: _____
_____
_____
_____
_____
_____
_____
_____

Date: _____ Appointment with: _____

Reason for visit: _____

_____

Notes: _____

_____

_____

_____

_____

_____

_____

_____

_____

Date: _____ Appointment with: _____

Reason for visit: _____

_____

Notes: _____

_____

_____

_____

_____

_____

_____

_____

Date: _____ Appointment with: _____

Reason for visit: _____
_____

Notes: _____
_____
_____
_____
_____
_____
_____
_____
_____

Date: _____ Appointment with: _____

Reason for visit: _____
_____

Notes: _____
_____
_____
_____
_____
_____
_____
_____

Date: _____ Appointment with: _____

Reason for visit: _____

_____

Notes: _____

_____

_____

_____

_____

_____

_____

_____

_____

Date: _____ Appointment with: _____

Reason for visit: _____

_____

Notes: _____

_____

_____

_____

_____

_____

_____

_____

Date: _____ Appointment with: _____

Reason for visit: _____
_____

Notes: _____
_____
_____
_____
_____
_____
_____
_____

Date: _____ Appointment with: _____

Reason for visit: _____
_____

Notes: _____
_____
_____
_____
_____
_____
_____

Date: _____ Appointment with: _____

Reason for visit: _____

_____

Notes: _____

_____

_____

_____

_____

_____

_____

_____

_____

* * *

Date: _____ Appointment with: _____

Reason for visit: _____

_____

Notes: _____

_____

_____

_____

_____

_____

_____

_____

Date: _____ Appointment with: _____

Reason for visit: _____

_____

Notes: _____

_____

_____

_____

_____

_____

_____

_____

_____

Date: _____ Appointment with: _____

Reason for visit: _____

_____

Notes: _____

_____

_____

_____

_____

_____

_____

_____

Date: _____ Appointment with: _____

Reason for visit: _____
_____

Notes: _____
_____
_____
_____
_____
_____
_____
_____
_____

Date: _____ Appointment with: _____

Reason for visit: _____
_____

Notes: _____
_____
_____
_____
_____
_____
_____
_____

Date: _____ Appointment with: _____

Reason for visit: _____
_____

Notes: _____
_____
_____
_____
_____
_____
_____
_____

Date: _____ Appointment with: _____

Reason for visit: _____
_____

Notes: _____
_____
_____
_____
_____
_____
_____
_____

Date: _____ Appointment with: _____

Reason for visit: _____

_____

Notes: _____

_____

_____

_____

_____

_____

_____

_____

_____

Date: _____ Appointment with: _____

Reason for visit: _____

_____

Notes: _____

_____

_____

_____

_____

_____

_____

_____

Date: _____ Appointment with: _____

Reason for visit: _____
_____

Notes: _____
_____
_____
_____
_____
_____
_____
_____
_____

Date: _____ Appointment with: _____

Reason for visit: _____
_____

Notes: _____
_____
_____
_____
_____
_____
_____
_____

Date: _____ Appointment with: _____

Reason for visit: _____
_____

Notes: _____
_____
_____
_____
_____
_____
_____
_____

Date: _____ Appointment with: _____

Reason for visit: _____
_____

Notes: _____
_____
_____
_____
_____
_____
_____

Date: _____ Appointment with: _____

Reason for visit: _____
_____

Notes: _____
_____
_____
_____
_____
_____
_____
_____
_____

Date: _____ Appointment with: _____

Reason for visit: _____
_____

Notes: _____
_____
_____
_____
_____
_____
_____
_____

Date: _____ Appointment with: _____

Reason for visit: _____
_____

Notes: _____
_____
_____
_____
_____
_____
_____
_____
_____
_____

Date: _____ Appointment with: _____

Reason for visit: _____
_____

Notes: _____
_____
_____
_____
_____
_____
_____
_____

Date: _____ Appointment with: _____

Reason for visit: _____

_____

Notes: _____

_____

_____

_____

_____

_____

_____

_____

_____

Date: _____ Appointment with: _____

Reason for visit: _____

_____

Notes: _____

_____

_____

_____

_____

_____

_____

_____

HOSPITALIZATIONS

Hospitalization For: _____

Admission Date: _____ Hospital: _____

Doctor(s):_____
_____
_____

Reason for Hospitalization: _____
_____
_____
_____
_____
_____
_____
_____

Discharge Date: _____

Discharge Instructions:_____
_____
_____
_____
_____
_____
_____
_____
_____
_____
_____
_____

Hospitalizations

Hospitalization For: _____

Admission Date: _____ Hospital: _____

Doctor(s):_____
_____
_____

Reason for Hospitalization: _____
_____
_____
_____
_____
_____
_____

Discharge Date: _____

Discharge Instructions:_____
_____
_____
_____
_____
_____
_____
_____
_____
_____
_____
_____
_____

HOSPITALIZATIONS

Hospitalization For: _____

Admission Date: _____ Hospital: _____

Doctor(s):_____
_____
_____

Reason for Hospitalization: _____
_____
_____
_____
_____
_____
_____
_____

Discharge Date: _____

Discharge Instructions:_____
_____
_____
_____
_____
_____
_____
_____
_____
_____
_____
_____

Hospitalizations

Hospitalization For: _____

Admission Date: _____ Hospital: _____

Doctor(s): _____

_____

_____

Reason for Hospitalization: _____

_____

_____

_____

_____

_____

_____

Discharge Date: _____

Discharge Instructions: _____

_____

_____

_____

_____

_____

_____

_____

_____

_____

_____

_____

HOSPITALIZATIONS

Hospitalization For: _____

Admission Date: _____ Hospital: _____

Doctor(s):_____
_____
_____

Reason for Hospitalization: _____
_____
_____
_____
_____
_____
_____

Discharge Date: _____

Discharge Instructions:_____
_____
_____
_____
_____
_____
_____
_____
_____
_____
_____

HOSPITALIZATIONS

Hospitalization For: _____

Admission Date: _____ Hospital: _____

Doctor(s):_____

_____

_____

Reason for Hospitalization: _____

_____

_____

_____

_____

_____

_____

_____

Discharge Date: _____

Discharge Instructions:_____

_____

_____

_____

_____

_____

_____

_____

_____

_____

_____

HOSPITALIZATIONS

Hospitalization For: _____

Admission Date: _____ Hospital: _____

Doctor(s): _____
_____
_____

Reason for Hospitalization: _____
_____
_____
_____
_____
_____
_____
_____

Discharge Date: _____

Discharge Instructions: _____
_____
_____
_____
_____
_____
_____
_____
_____
_____
_____
_____

HOSPITALIZATIONS

Hospitalization For: _____

Admission Date: _____ Hospital: _____

Doctor(s):_____

_____

_____

Reason for Hospitalization: _____

_____

_____

_____

_____

_____

_____

_____

Discharge Date: _____

Discharge Instructions:_____

_____

_____

_____

_____

_____

_____

_____

_____

_____

_____

_____

HOSPITALIZATIONS

Hospitalization For: _____

Admission Date: _____ Hospital: _____

Doctor(s): _____
_____
_____

Reason for Hospitalization: _____
_____
_____
_____
_____
_____
_____

Discharge Date: _____

Discharge Instructions: _____
_____
_____
_____
_____
_____
_____
_____
_____
_____
_____
_____

HOSPITALIZATIONS

Hospitalization For: _____

Admission Date: _____ Hospital: _____

Doctor(s):_____

_____

_____

Reason for Hospitalization: _____

_____

_____

_____

_____

_____

_____

Discharge Date: _____

Discharge Instructions:_____

_____

_____

_____

_____

_____

_____

_____

_____

_____

_____

_____

HOSPITALIZATIONS

Hospitalization For: _____

Admission Date: _____ Hospital: _____

Doctor(s):_____
_____
_____

Reason for Hospitalization: _____
_____
_____
_____
_____
_____
_____

Discharge Date: _____

Discharge Instructions:_____
_____
_____
_____
_____
_____
_____
_____
_____
_____
_____
_____

Hospitalizations

Hospitalization For: _____

Admission Date: _____ Hospital: _____

Doctor(s):_____

_____

_____

Reason for Hospitalization: _____

_____

_____

_____

_____

_____

_____

Discharge Date: _____

Discharge Instructions:_____

_____

_____

_____

_____

_____

_____

_____

_____

_____

_____

_____

HOSPITALIZATIONS

Hospitalization For: _____

Admission Date: _____ Hospital: _____

Doctor(s): _____
_____
_____

Reason for Hospitalization: _____
_____
_____
_____
_____
_____
_____
_____

Discharge Date: _____

Discharge Instructions: _____
_____
_____
_____
_____
_____
_____
_____
_____
_____
_____
_____
_____

HOSPITALIZATIONS

Hospitalization For: _____

Admission Date: _____ Hospital: _____

Doctor(s):_____
_____
_____

Reason for Hospitalization: _____
_____
_____
_____
_____
_____
_____

Discharge Date: _____

Discharge Instructions:_____
_____
_____
_____
_____
_____
_____
_____
_____
_____
_____

HOSPITALIZATIONS

Hospitalization For: _____

Admission Date: _____ Hospital: _____

Doctor(s):_____
_____
_____

Reason for Hospitalization: _____
_____
_____
_____
_____
_____
_____

Discharge Date: _____

Discharge Instructions:_____
_____
_____
_____
_____
_____
_____
_____
_____
_____
_____
_____

HOSPITALIZATIONS

Hospitalization For: _____

Admission Date: _____ Hospital: _____

Doctor(s):_____
_____
_____

Reason for Hospitalization: _____
_____
_____
_____
_____
_____
_____

Discharge Date: _____

Discharge Instructions:_____
_____
_____
_____
_____
_____
_____
_____
_____
_____
_____
_____

HOSPITALIZATIONS

Hospitalization For: _____

Admission Date: _____ Hospital: _____

Doctor(s):_____

_____

_____

Reason for Hospitalization: _____

_____

_____

_____

_____

_____

_____

_____

Discharge Date: _____

Discharge Instructions:_____

_____

_____

_____

_____

_____

_____

_____

_____

_____

_____

_____

HOSPITALIZATIONS

Hospitalization For: _____

Admission Date: _____ Hospital: _____

Doctor(s): _____
_____
_____

Reason for Hospitalization: _____
_____
_____
_____
_____
_____
_____
_____

Discharge Date: _____

Discharge Instructions:_____
_____
_____
_____
_____
_____
_____
_____
_____
_____
_____
_____
_____

HOSPITALIZATIONS

Hospitalization For: _____

Admission Date: _____ Hospital: _____

Doctor(s): _____
_____
_____

Reason for Hospitalization: _____
_____
_____
_____
_____
_____
_____

Discharge Date: _____

Discharge Instructions: _____
_____
_____
_____
_____
_____
_____
_____
_____
_____
_____
_____

HOSPITALIZATIONS

Hospitalization For: _____

Admission Date: _____ Hospital: _____

Doctor(s):_____
_____
_____

Reason for Hospitalization: _____
_____
_____
_____
_____
_____
_____

Discharge Date: _____

Discharge Instructions:_____
_____
_____
_____
_____
_____
_____
_____
_____
_____
_____
_____

TREATMENT PLAN

Treatment Plan For: _____

Treatment Start Date: _____ Treatment End Date: _____

Treatment Type: _____
_____
_____

Doctor(s): _____
_____
_____

Treatment Facility: _____
_____
_____

Treatment Prescribed: _____
_____
_____
_____
_____
_____
_____
_____

Results: _____
_____
_____
_____
_____

✴ TREATMENT PLAN

Treatment Plan For: _____

Treatment Start Date: _____ Treatment End Date: _____

Treatment Type: _____
_____
_____

Doctor(s):_____
_____
_____

Treatment Facility: _____
_____
_____

Treatment Prescribed: _____
_____
_____
_____
_____
_____
_____
_____
_____

Results: _____
_____
_____
_____
_____

✹ TREATMENT PLAN

Treatment Plan For: _____

Treatment Start Date: _____Treatment End Date: _____

Treatment Type: _____

_____

_____

Doctor(s):_____

_____

_____

Treatment Facility: _____

_____

_____

Treatment Prescribed: _____

_____

_____

_____

_____

_____

_____

_____

_____

Results: _____

_____

_____

_____

_____

TREATMENT PLAN

Treatment Plan For: _____

Treatment Start Date: _____ Treatment End Date: _____

Treatment Type: _____
_____
_____

Doctor(s): _____
_____
_____

Treatment Facility: _____
_____
_____

Treatment Prescribed: _____
_____
_____
_____
_____
_____
_____
_____
_____

Results: _____
_____
_____
_____
_____

✦ Treatment Plan

Treatment Plan For: _____

Treatment Start Date: _____ Treatment End Date: _____

Treatment Type: _____
_____
_____

Doctor(s): _____
_____
_____

Treatment Facility: _____
_____
_____

Treatment Prescribed: _____
_____
_____
_____
_____
_____
_____
_____
_____

Results: _____
_____
_____
_____
_____

TREATMENT PLAN

Treatment Plan For: _____

Treatment Start Date: _____ Treatment End Date: _____

Treatment Type: _____
_____
_____

Doctor(s): _____
_____
_____

Treatment Facility: _____
_____
_____

Treatment Prescribed: _____
_____
_____
_____
_____
_____
_____
_____
_____

Results: _____
_____
_____
_____
_____

HEALTH CARE PROVIDERS AND ADDITIONAL RESOURCES

	Name	Contact Information
Caregivers/ Nurses		
Home Health:		
Occupational Therapists:		
Physical Therapists:		
Respiratory Therapists:		
Speech Therapists:		
Rehabilitation Centers:		

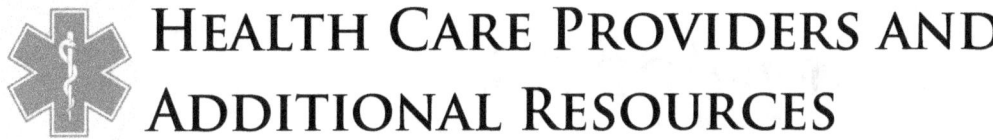

HEALTH CARE PROVIDERS AND ADDITIONAL RESOURCES

	Name	Contact Information
Medical Transports:	_____	_____
	_____	_____
Veteran's Administration:	_____	_____
	_____	_____
Medicare:	_____	_____
	_____	_____
Medicaid:	_____	_____
	_____	_____
Social Security Administration:	_____	_____
	_____	_____
Pastor/Church/ Church Groups:	_____	_____
	_____	_____
	_____	_____
	_____	_____
Medical Alert Systems:	_____	_____
	_____	_____
Medical Equipment And Supplies:	_____	_____
	_____	_____
	_____	_____
Hospice:	_____	_____
	_____	_____

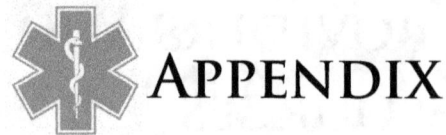# APPENDIX

Attach documentation such as Living Will, Power of Attorney, Durable Healthcare Power of Attorney, Power of Attorney for a Child, Advance Directives, copy of Insurance Cards, etc.

- _____
- _____
- _____
- _____
- _____
- _____
- _____
- _____
- _____
- _____
- _____
- _____
- _____